What's A Parent To Do

A Guide to Raising a Successful Young Adult

Carolyn Hildebrandt

CONTENTS

FOREWORD

Being a parent is hard but trying to be a good parent is even harder. My dear friend Carolyn, has always had a deep passion for helping support parents in their times of struggle with their children. Her many decades of experience, her educational research and study, and her volunteer work shows her commitment to this work. Parenting, I would argue, is one of the toughest jobs out there. This book was written out of love for parents who need support, encouragement, and no-none-sensical advice and some tough love (from time to time) while trying to love, protect, discipline and communicate with their child. The content in this book will help you focus on simple, small actions and behaviors that add up to consistent behaviors and life and relationship patterns with a teenager struggling to come to terms with a life. Carolyn helps to humanize what teenagers are going through and why they act out or behave the way they do at times with kindness, humility and compassion but also consistency, firmness and transparency. I would encourage any and all parents to read this book, reflect and think of ways we can all grow in our parenting. I don't know one parent, who would not look back at their relationship with their child, and not want to change something or have a do-over at times. We grow with our children in parenting and this book will help you take those steps with intention and love.

Dr. Natalie L. Tucker
Vice President and Academic Dean
Marian University Ancilla College

Dr. Natalie Tucker has worked at Marian University Ancilla College (MUAC) for the past 3 years as the Associate Professor of Agriculture and Department Head and currently, as the Dean of Academics and Vice President of MUAC. She worked for Ancilla College as an adjunct faculty member for 7 years teaching agriculture and sciences. She is the owner of NLD Contractual Services in which she provides court program development, specialty court program development, and grant writing. Prior, she also worked for Purdue University for 12 years in the role of academic advising and teaching in the College of Agriculture and as a Purdue Extension Director and 4-H Youth Development Educator in Pulaski County. She obtained a Bachelor of Science in Agricultural Communication; a Masters of Arts in American History; and Doctoral Degree in Agriculture all from

Purdue University.   She is a wife and mother to 3 busy children and loves to travel, read, learn and run.

WHAT'S A PARENT TO DO

A Guide to Raising a Successful Young Adult

INTRODUCTION

This book is focused at leading you through the process of re-training your child to become a more disciplined teen-ager and one who is interested in school and one that understands the importance of such a task. I have laid it out in a manner in which you can follow as a guide. The many parents and students I have recommended these steps to, who have completed them, have experienced success. It is my intention to aid you in the process of getting your student back on track. This will be one of the most challenging tasks you have undertaken in your life. Just the mere fact that you are reading this book means your looking for solutions to existing challenges you are facing with your child or you think you are headed in the wrong direction and you are trying to avoid this detour in life. Whatever your reason for picking up this little book I commend you. You are being brave in loving your child and wanting to support them in their future success.

OK, let's get started.

CHAPTER ONE

First, there are numerous types of problems you might be encountering as the parent of a teenager or even a pre-teen. Now that's a broad range. That will take care of any age from seven – nineteen. Listed below are a few major problems I have come in contact with as an Academic Advisor at a middle school, high school and University.

1. Students making "D's" and "F's"
2. Student not attending classes
3. Student truant from school
4. Student lying
5. Student deleting unfavorable emails
Usually from the school to the parent
6. Student being defiant with authority

Unfortunately, most of the students and parents I see are experiencing some measure of difficulty with each other, their student and perhaps even the school.

There are many remedies for each problem listed above. Each solution is like being given medication by your doctor, unless you take the medication it will not provide you with the healing agents your body and mind need in order to heal you. The same is true with a number of bad habits. This process will need both your commitment and your child's commitment. Unless your child buys into the process to change established habits, it will never work. Of all the advice I will give you throughout this book, the very best advice I, or anyone else, will give you is to make sure your child is willing to participate in the plan you are setting forth. By including them in the plan you are showing them trust and love. It is very discouraging to meet with parents and they do not want their teenager to be present. They may enter my office and I ask where the child is and they say, "we wanted to talk to you alone." This is indeed a good idea if you are going into intense therapy. However, when you are going to get advice on what direction your student needs to go in school it's best to have your student with you. Whether this is a plan to get them into college, get them married, learn to brush their teeth or learn personal hygiene they must be a part of the decision-making process. They must see they, too, have control. This will establish respect as well as give them the feeling they are somewhat in charge of their own life. We all want to be in control of what happens to us in life. Young people are no different. They must feel they are in control of their destiny.

Now, don't go off the deep end here and say, "Now you're in middle school or high school so I will let you take care of yourself. You must learn to be responsible." In fact, these young people are probably more confused now than when they entered kindergarten. This is part of brain development. At least when they entered kindergarten, they knew YOU were in charge and YOU were going to take care of them. Now, they're just not sure who is in charge, or for that matter, who is supposed to be in charge. In their small brains and big bodies, they get confused and say to themselves, "I look like an adult, I talk like an adult, I walk like an adult, therefore, I must be an adult." Wrong!!! Not only are they confused mentally and emotionally, they are confused physically. Their hormones are raging. Mom, you think you had problems when you were carrying them, well they are experiencing some of the same hormonal imbalance you experienced, only in a different way. The young boys are starting to think about their bodies. The young girls' bodies are changing dramatically. Dreams are in the boy's head. The girls are wearing things they have never dreamed of wearing nor wanted to wear. Teachers are pulling at them to act a certain way, "grow up, behave, do homework, so on and so on." Threats of failure loom all around. *"If you don't do well in school, you won't do well in life." "What's wrong with you?" "Are you stupid?"* Yes, these are things that are being said to them. Even social media pressures are coming at them constantly. Sometimes I think it's a miracle any of these kids make it today, and you know what, most make it and make it well.

No one factor is the answer to difficult situations. Sometimes many different methods must be tried in order to resolve issues that rise up and slap us in the face. Do not be afraid to take the big step to develop a method of resolution for your particular situation. I hope when you finish this book you will have a better grip on life with your child and that you will have learned that peace, confidence and success can be obtained even when living with a teenager.

CHAPTER TWO

We live in a quick fix world today. We get our dinner from a drive through window, our lunch on the go at a food court, and talk or text on our cell phones for most communications. We are always connected to something or someone at a distance. It is no wonder that when our teenagers begin having problems, we call the school and say, "Hey, fix this problem with my child." Oops, things just do not happen that fast in the real world. Once a parent called me to tell me I should call her son in to make sure he is doing his homework. I explained to her that is why it is called homework because it is done at home and hopefully the parents supervise to see that it is completed in the correct way.

One of the most important things we are missing in our lives today is true realism. We sit our children down to do homework or send them to their room and trust they are, in fact, doing homework. Then we rush them off to take their baths and get ready for bed. Most of the time we fail to really sit with them to go over their work or ask them questions pertaining to that history assignment, or math assignment or English assignment. We do not routinely talk to our children about school. Due to our own busy schedules, we want them to be independent so we do not have to follow up on the details of their assignments. Many times, we are more concerned with the soccer game, dance lesson, cheerleader practice or the big game coming up on Friday night. It is our job, as a parent, to direct them to academic success first. We need to convey the message to our children that they are important and that we are interested in their academic success which will eventually lead to life success. We set the example. Young people need to see us using our leisure time in a productive manner in order to set the example. Try to find a special interest that your student has and stay informed about it so you can talk to them about what they are interested in. Maybe this is a sport, skateboarding, cars, or surfing. This is a familiar one to me since I lived in Southern California for 13 years during the time my own three children were in school and the beach was a mere two miles from the high school I worked at. Perhaps your student is interested in computers or gaming. Whatever their interest, find out something about it so you can talk to them on a level that shows you do care about things they are interested in other than *school.* You will be amazed to see them respond to you. Think about it, if you have someone who can talk to you about something you are interested in, don't you respond? Of course, you do and so will your child. Try it! What have you got to lose?

We have heard the old saying that we need to be a friend to our children. A friend they can confide in, a friend they can be truly honest with. However, our children need to see us as a parent first. They need us to be a role model. This means a person in charge, the boss, giving out the agenda of the day. They are not the ones that have to plan the family routine. They are the ones that have to continue to grow, learn, and participate in life in order to survive successfully. This is how it should be. Parents are parents and have the final say in what will and what will not be done. Are children here to just say, "Yes Ma'am" and "Yes sir"? That is a concept that simply does not work. Children are here to develop and become productive adults contributing to society and adding love and appreciation for life. Absolutely, children must learn to show respect and to set boundaries in order to develop into the kind of adult we all hope for. We are here to guide them along that path.

We, as parents, must find the path to be parent and friend. The official definition of the word friend is, "a person who has a strong liking for and trust in another." https://www.meriamwebster.com. This is certainly a goal we all desire to be realized in our relationship with our children and still hold the authority and respect as a parent.

As parents, you must learn to change your hat many times in a day, from parent to friend to disciplinary and back to parent again. Children must see we mean what we say, and say what we mean. They must see us living our own lives in a manner that is consistent with our words.

In the following process you will learn a very important lesson which is, if you do not carry through with what you say, don't even consider trying to put it in place. Kids are the sharpest things you will ever encounter. They have a memory like an elephant. They learn quickly whether you are a push over or a General, "Mom means what she says," or "Dad means what he says." You, as the parent, set the stage when they are about one or two years of age. So, at this point, if you have not been following through with your statements you better get ready for a dramatic tug of war. Realize that your teenager has already learned some initial cue words that you normally use like, "I mean it," One of my favorites is, "I'm counting to five." I used this one many times with my own three children. It never works. You know if we have laid out the rules of the game to the child why would we have to count to five before we take action. Is this a baseball game where three strikes and you're out? No, it is a life pattern.

Healthy patterns may look like some of the following:

    Parents going to work everyday
    Parents keeping the house in order
    Dinner being served every night
    Lunches being prepared every morning
    Laundry being done in a timely manner

Simply stated – a disciplined life

CHAPTER THREE

Getting started is the easy part. When do you get started? How do you start? Where do you start?

WHEN – Now

WHERE – At Home

HOW- Little by Little

We know we have already missed the first two steps because we now have a teenager and we are looking for help. Just know it is not too late to follow through with the third step, HOW. Little by Little – that is how Rome was built so surely it will work for building a life of good habits and realizing successful skills for living for our children.

The first rule is to sit down and have a meeting or serious talk with your child. Schedule a definite time to talk to your child. Schedule a time when younger siblings are in bed or they are being taken care of in order that the two of you can talk without interruptions. Make sure the phone can be turned off or answered by someone else. When you are in the middle of a meaningful conversation with your child you do not want to stop to answer a call even if it seems to be a very important call. This interruption will cause the line of communication and connection between you and your child to be lost. Believe me, teenagers can be the most offended people in the world for the most inconsequential reason. They truly believe the world evolves around them and if they are already doing poorly with life skills answering that phone or any other interruption that takes you away from this moment will be used by them against you. This interruption will serve as their scapegoat. I have often heard students complain that, "Mom doesn't listen to me, she is always talking or texting on the phone." Or "Mom is always running off to see what my little sister or brother is doing." I know you are not always on the phone but remember we are trying to look at things from their angle. When a person feels they have failed in some area they will grasp at any reason for justification for their behavior. This is exactly what your child is feeling and doing. Their perception of what is happening is real to them even though you may have a completely different perception. This is normal. None of us want to recognize the fact that we have failed in any way. You are probably feeling some of the same emotions your child is feeling.

The key here is to know you are in charge, even though right now they are calling the shots. This is a learned behavior and you and your child are now beginning to learn a new behavior. Be very specific when you plan this talk. Tell your child exactly what time and place you are going to sit and discuss the issues facing you both. When you say, "we are going to talk tonight at 8:00 PM" be ready. Do not be a minute late for the appointed time. This is the time you are setting new rules and expectations. These expectations are not just for your child, they are for both of you. Tell them your goal is to see their grades improving, see them truly studying and applying themselves to achieve in school and thus life. Let me assure you they are expecting to see you follow through with every single word you say. When you are specific with the plan, the new rules, the new expectations your teen is more likely to buy into this plan of action. They will not go peacefully and they will be looking for an escape route. It will be up to you to be prepared for any and every unexpected attempt they may have to escape.

During the conversation you will need to deal with exact issues at hand, poor grades, skipping class, not completing assignments and any additional issues that have come up. Make a list prior to your meeting in order to ensure all areas of concern are addressed and dealt with in order that you do not have to come back later and say, "... and one more thing..." This will stir up feelings of hopelessness in your child and has the potential to cause your child to dismiss the importance of the situation.

Take a direct approach on each issue. Excuses are not allowed in this meeting. Each time a reason or excuse is offered for something not being done simply say, "that's fine, but from this moment on we are going to do differently." Stress the "WE" here. Remind your child that you intend to be an active part of this process. Tell them you completely understand this was obviously too much responsibility for them and now you are here to help them learn a new method and acquire better habits. Be sincere, if you over exaggerate or lack sincerity in your understanding of their situation your child will only become angry with you. The manner in which you respond is extremely important. It is best to try and agree with your child on as many issues as possible during this meeting. Then explain the new direction both of you are going to take. An example of a response could be, "Yes, you are right your teacher is one of the hardest in this subject, however, I know you are capable of meeting their requirements for this class." You have agreed with them and stated your confidence in their ability to achieve success. Your goal at this point is to build a relationship with your child and establish a bond of trust and cooperation. You are building a partnership; you are helping them understand what is happening. You are letting them know you are on their side and letting them know you love them and will stand by them as they learn new methods and change behaviors and attitudes.

CHAPTER FOUR

It is important for us to take a look at the whole picture at this point. You do not want to be doing this just to say you have tried everything possible and nothing works. Many parents I have met with sometimes start our conversations with these very words, "I have tried everything possible and nothing works." It may indeed seem as though you have tried everything, however, I assure you the word "everything" will need to be redefined. I myself, have used this phrase and ended my statement with, "I don't know what to do?" or "What's a parent to do?" The truth was I had only tried everything for a short time. I stress the word short. In fact, I had tried "everything" for only a few days with no measure of consistency. Consistency is the key. This is another hard part I have been telling you about. Not only has your child learned inconsistent patterns of life, so have we. They have to know your support will not change this time. Don't give up!

Your next step is yet another big step in the direction you want to go. This will require a great deal of effort and time and the "patience of Job". The patience of Job refers to remaining patient and calm to do what must be done even in the face of insurmountable problems, pressures or disturbances occurring at this time, www.biblestudytools.com   I must warn you this could have a tremendous impact on the physical and mental health of our child if you half-heartedly undertake this step. They could become extremely angry if you fail to uphold your end of the new commitment you have agreed upon, just as you might become angry if they fail to uphold their part of the bargain. They may change their eating patterns or they may just ignore you which will lead to an array of other issues to deal with. You will jeopardize losing their respect and trust if you give up and say one thing and do another. You must always be reminding yourself that you are the adult and they are the child. You cannot afford to let your emotions compromise any situation you find yourself in. There will be times you have to hold it together to deal with a situation and then go in another room, bury your head in a pillow and just scream. Then pull yourself together and come out with a smile of confidence and assurance on your face. Trust me, your child will notice!

A parent came in my office one day and poured out his story of extreme difficulties in his home with his 15-year-old daughter. It was a sad story involving more than just bad grades. She began hanging out with a "bad" group of older kids. Her outfits she wore changed, her make-up changed and most importantly her total attitude changed and all for the worse. In the course of the conversation, he shared that he had told his teenager he was throwing her clothes out the window and kicking her out of the house. This would have been ok in extreme situations, except the child was only 15. By law parents are responsible for their children until 18. This shows us we have to be very careful with what we state to our children. Make sure you can truly follow through with any consequence you state is going to happen. I have found teenagers know the laws better than you or I do. Keep your threats of consequences to a minimum. Think through your plan of action. State that you are going to contact the teacher or teachers, then contact that teacher or all six teachers. State that you are going to check their homework, then check that homework. Do not let one night go by where you say, "OK, if you are sure, you have everything done, I'll take your word for it tonight. I better not find out that you didn't finish all of your assignments." You have just taken 100 steps backwards. This is what commitment is all about. I know you are tired. I know you are frustrated. I know you want a few minutes to yourself. Not Now! Get in there and check that homework, all of it. Help your child redo that math problem. Call out those spelling words, economic terms, or whatever it is they are assigned to learn. It will take a little while to see progress, but you will see progress. When you are faithful, results will be realized. The rewards will be seeing the change in your child as they realize they can indeed do this.

Develop an active plan you both can live with. This will take time and a great deal of effort. You must first have a collaborative plan of action for you and your child to ensure success. Without a plan you can build on do not expect change to occur. With a plan you can build anything. With a plan you and your child will be successful.

Your plan must be the foundation on which you will begin making changes in behavior, in habits, in attitude and so much more.

CHAPTER FIVE

The first part of your plan will be the foundation. This will include the time and place for homework. In addition, you must specify the nights homework will be done. I recommend Monday through Thursday. This gives both of you the week-end off and a break from the intensity of revamping your lives. I used to ground my children Monday through Friday in order that we could all have a break. When you ground your child, you are also grounding yourself.

The schedule could look something like this:

<u>Days of the week</u>	<u>Hours</u>
Monday – Thursday	7:00 – 8:30
Friday – Sunday	No assigned study time
	(unless special assignment from teacher)

I would not recommend saying they can do whatever they want to Friday through Sunday. That statement could come back to cause problems for later on. Many times, family occasions or special events come up. You do not want your child to come back to you saying, "I don't want to go to grandma's house, YOU SAID, I could do whatever I want to do on the week-ends and I want to go out with my friends." This is a situation you want to protect yourself from.

Be aware and make sure your child is aware that there may be days homework will have to be done on a Saturday or Sunday night. Teachers occasionally will schedule a big test for Monday morning. This is completely normal and helps prepare our children for life as an adult. Getting our children ready to go out in the real world and face the good, the bad and the challenging situations and the responsibilities of life is our goal. Once students learn that a teacher is not being "mean" when they assign homework for the week-end, they will be making great strides in accepting the responsibility of school and life.

The second part of your plan should be to determine how this hour and a half will be spent studying. Yes, indeed, there are many ways students' study. Some look at a pencil for the allotted time. Some dream of what they are going to do as soon as they move out of "your" house or just wonder how long it is going to take before you are going to stop pushing this study time stuff. They are pretty confident you will not last because perhaps they have experienced short periods of the same thing in the past. Your goal here will be to remain calm as you explain to your child that homework will be done and you simply stand firm. Assure them things will be different this time. Perhaps you have attempted a similar approach in the past but were unable to follow through until the final goal had been achieved. This is what they are thinking about and feel confident this time will simply be a repeat of the past.

The third part of your plan will be setting boundaries for study time. Boundaries may look like this:

NO MUSIC

NO PHONE

NO TELEVISION

NO GAMING

NO SURFING THE COMPUTER OR OTHER DEVICES

In the beginning this will be an enormous shock for your child. Just the idea of no music for some teenagers is almost more than they can handle. It is important to realize that they are only spending an hour to an hour and a half on homework. We are developing good study habits. I stress the "WE" here because you are definitely an integral part of this process. When and if the phone rings, it can simply go to messages or better yet, just turn the phone off for this period of time. I have found that if a student answers their phone during this designated time their minds will not return to their studies. The remainder of the study time will be spent with a wandering mind where their thoughts shift away from the task before them. They will be recalling what was discussed with their friend, where they are going this weekend or about the upcoming sports event. Anything but the homework they are supposed to be doing. Be prepared, your child will give you all manner of reasons they must take a call. Such as: Just this once, they must talk to their friend because his friends Dad is leaving for Alaska tomorrow and he has to get his only set of gym clothes he left with his friend. The best excuse I have heard is if you keep them from taking this call you will surely ruin their life forever, and there will be no need for them to ever study again because "YOU" have caused irreparable damage for any chance of them getting into college. Don't forget, you are the PARENT, and parent is in capital letters. Whatever is happening in the outside world during this hour and a half will wait. Their only opportunity for happiness will not, forever, pass them by.

This practice will be difficult for a few days or perhaps a few weeks. Sometimes breaking into a new pattern of study or anything new in life is extremely difficult. Hang in there, things will get better and adjustments in attitude will improve.

Music, will be the real challenge. What can possibly be the logic for not having their earbuds? Don't you know they can study better with music on? A favorite statement is, "Mom, I can't think when it's so quiet." The music must be off or your student will not be able to think or retain anything they are studying. In the case that some type of music must be on and you make a compromise with your child just tell them it will have to be classical music. That will certainly give them a jolt. Most will respond with statements such as, "Yuck! I can't listen to that." Many professionals believe listening to classical music can provide intellectual stimulation by boosting memory, concentration and creative thinking. *https://interlude.hk*

Perhaps all students should be required to listen to classical music before taking a test. In reality, I have had students who actually learned to like listening to classical music. I required my own children to do this and they still listen to classical music today, they are in their 40's and my sons have become successful adults.

The no television, no gaming, no computer, no cell phones, news or TikTok time is quite simple and most students can comprehend this one without much trouble. Actually, the cable company has helped us out here, in that, there are not many things today's young people like to watch anyway. In the event there is something your child wants to watch no problem. The invention of the new technology allows us the opportunity to record a program and watch it at a later time. Problem solved.

As I stated previously, this new routine might present some real challenges to you and your child. Due to the difficulties in learning a new behavior you may have to break this hour and a half up into smaller segments, 15 or 20 minutes at a time. Unfortunately, teenagers, for the most part do not have a long attention span. Therefore, you might need to fine tune this study time. When you break the study time in segments this gives the student time to get up, walk around, go to the bathroom and get a snack. This will not allow time to call a friend. Remember what I said about that phone. Be aware your child might try your commitment to this new program. Stay strong and committed to your word.

Another main element in your plan will be attendance in school. Many times, when students are facing challenges in school, they are also facing challenges in attendance.   Schools are designed to be attended. Teachers set up their classroom curriculum and grading system incorporating a percentage of the grade coming from classroom participation. Students who are not present in the classroom receive zeros on this portion of the grade.

Most middle schools and high schools have an attendance accounting system. As a parent you need to make sure you know your child's school attendance policy. I highly recommend you contact the attendance secretary or one of the administrators to explain exactly how their system works. Then and only then will you be able to take issue with your child. Once again, remember you are the parent and you must be completely informed on technical issues like this rather than relay on what your child is telling you. When your child says, "I don't know why that teacher marked me absent, I swear I was in class." You can respond with an intelligent, informed answer like, "I know why the teacher marked you absent..." Once your student realizes they can no longer get away with telling you what they think you want to hear rather than the truth they will begin to conform to the rules laid forth by you and by the school. Not only does your child need to be in class to achieve academic success they need to be prepared and willing to be engaged within the classroom.

As homework starts getting done, and studying becomes a routine each night, classroom participation usually follows, homework is completed as assigned and grades begin to go up. Students know the answers and they want to share that knowledge. They begin to feel self-assured and many times are amazed at how much they have actually learned. I have never seen a student that is turning his school habits around come in my office all down hearted and ashamed of their success. They come in excited, "Mrs. H., I'm doing great! My teacher says I have brought my grades up and it really does feel good." Truly this is their response. They begin to get hooked on pride in themselves rather than resigned to failure. No one wants to fail. Human nature is geared to achieving goals and producing. What we are trying to do is show these young people that producing something good is worthwhile and immensely rewarding.

Set your ground rules when you set your plan up. That way, there will be no questions or misunderstandings as to what is expected. I have seen this plan work many times with students I have advised over my 10 years in a middle school and high school.

I had one student who was going into his senior year who was very concerned about passing his final required class in order to graduate. I admit, I was quite concerned myself. He had spent the past three years of high school barely getting "D's" with a few "C's" and "B's" thrown in. He had gone to summer school every summer to make up required classes for graduation. Now, he was entering his senior year and he had a teacher who was known for being a very challenging teacher for one of his major academic subjects. I told him exactly what to do. The same approach I have laid out for you. He followed through with each of the suggestions I gave him. He spent the hour and one-half each night studying, he turned in all his homework on time, he did extra preparation for tests, he was not only present every day for class, he participated in the discussions in class. He shared with me he didn't say much in class but he did raise his hand to volunteer answers during discussion time. He made a "B" in the class. He graduated high school on time and felt empowered to face the next phase of his life journey. He was so proud of his achievements and felt that unmistakable elation that only comes from doing something well. He had reached a new level of success.

CHAPTER SIX

It is extremely important for young people to learn that what they do today will determine what they are allowed to do tomorrow. A student who takes Algebra I and earns a "D" in the class will not be allowed to continue to Geometry or Algebra II. A student that earns a "C" in English I Honors, will not be recommended to take English II Honors. This is a life lesson that will stay with them forever. Each segment of school prepares students to proceed to the next segment successfully. As a result, when a student is experiencing challenges in school, they will certainly begin to feel less confident about themselves and many times fall further and further behind. Be aware, they also become experts on covering these negative feelings up. They begin to internalize feelings of being stupid, ugly, a failure, worthless and unloved because of their lack of success in school. Unsuccessful students become overwhelmed as they have not learned the basic skills of time management and study skills. Successful students learn to be optimistic about their pathways to academic success.

Think of their grades as their paychecks. When they are a dedicated student, they receive good grades. When they are undisciplined in school their grades reflect their lack of effort. The same impact happens in the workplace. When they are good workers, they receive a good wage and usually excel in whatever field they choose to pursue. When they are an employ who fails to fulfill the expectations or responsibilities of their job, they will surely struggle in the workplace just as they struggled in school. Many times, in advising students, when I parallel this simile students begin to understand and accept responsibilities for their performance.

Poor grades do not always reflect a useless worker. Sometimes students having difficulties in school is due to something out of their control like a learning disability that has not been identified or perhaps another type of learning problem. I explain to students that going to school is their job just like going to work is their parents' job. I don't always like going to work every day but I do like having a nice car to drive and going home to a nice home. When I choose not to work, I am making the choice to not have these things in my life. The same is true for them, if they choose not to be engaged in school and participate in their education, they are making the choice to not earn good grades. They are also making the choice to face more challenging situations going forward in life. As cruel as it seems, I tell students to go pick out a shopping cart and decide what color blanket they want because there is a good chance that is where they are headed, unless

Mom and Dad intend to support them the rest of their lives. Parents, you too need to be aware that this may be your future too.

Just as a student determines his future, so a parent determines their future by what they allow to occur today. It is very difficult to be "hard" on your child. We do everything in our power to make their lives easy. We want to believe them. We want to always think the best of them; However, this is not always possible. I would never call a child a liar. I would point out to them, that it appears evident, through their grades and comments from their teachers, they are not ready to handle the responsibility of school and all the demands and requirements being placed on them. Therefore, you are going to pick up the pieces and get them back on track. As the parent you must separate your perception from the reality you are living.

Self-esteem is how we value and perceive ourselves. Knowing how to set goals and achieve them, how you act and feel about yourself and others. Ones self-esteem can be difficult to change. Knowing one has worth impacts our emotional state and impacts our ability to triumph or fall into despair. It can produce pride or shame in how we feel and view ourselves. Students who are experiencing failure in school, generally have a low self-esteem. Low self-esteem makes it very difficult to value ourselves and impacts our abilities to succeed. This is why it is important to address these issues and resolve to improve on expectations. Keep in mind the expectations we are talking about are the ones they have for themselves as well as the ones we have for them. Believing you can be successful allows you to be open to receive success. Change isn't easy. You and your child are in the process of changing many years of unsuccessful habits. The two of you are swapping out bad habits for good habits. You are establishing healthy, more productive behaviors.

Parents, a very important fact to always keep in the front of your mind at this point is that if you are always screaming at your child to do this or do that, stop it. Stop it right now! Could you go to work every day and do a good job if your boss was screaming at you, looking down your neck to see what you were doing?   Of course not, neither can your child.

You have a plan in place. When to study, where to study, and now, how to study. The rules have been laid out. You do not have to scream anymore. As a matter of fact, when things are not being done according to schedule your voice should go lower, to almost a whisper. The softer your voice becomes the harder they will have to listen, especially if this is an unusual occurrence. Your family dynamics may have trained your child to tune you out. They know you are going to resort to screaming and making threats.   Fool them, don't scream, don't make threats. Talk softly and simply restate the rules. You can even pull out the contract or written agreement if you have put your plan in writing.

CHAPTER SEVEN

Develop specific study techniques to promote learning. Psychologists have proven even animals can be trained. Therefore, it would stand to reason, this higher, more intelligent life form, your child, can be trained. You might be familiar with *Pavlov's dogs.* In the 1890's classical conditioning was discovered for training dogs. *https://www.simplypsychology.* We are indeed training our children for success.

This step will involve developing new study habits as well as techniques for successfully completing assignments. Organization will be a key factor here. When students get organized, they begin to see the benefits and realize triumph. Study time must be in a quite environment. Students must be sure they have written down the correct homework assignment for the evening. Nothing can be more discouraging to a student who is already having difficulty than doing an hour's worth of the wrong assignment. Keeping a reminder binder or day planner will be invaluable for this task. Modern technology has given us the benefit of having access to assignments through the use of the internet. Your child must learn or rather relearn to keep detailed instructions for homework and upcoming assignments. Knowing and understanding what a teacher wants is a key to success. When I was in college, I got so excited when I read the essay question on a final exam. I wrote two pages and felt quite pleased with myself. When I got the exam back, I found out I had misread the question and wrote a beautiful essay to the wrong question. What a heartbreak! Students who are having difficulties in school sometimes assume they know what is going on and as a result get the entire assignment confused. Help your child understand there is nothing wrong with asking a teacher to explain something again. Don't be fooled, this will be an arduous task. One thing I suggest at this point is for you, the parent, to put in a call to the teacher for clarification on assignments. Many times, this can be done by accessing the teacher's email or assignment page usually found on the school's webpage.

Now, I know Johnny is in the 10th grade and he should stand on his own two feet. This is true; however, Johnny has not been given the tools to achieve this task successfully. Make things perfectly clear and non-threating. Let them know that you are going to help him get on the right course. Unfortunately, as a rule, when students do not turn in homework, nor study for tests, nor show up for assigned extra help teachers retreat and throw in the towel. Then when the first efforts are made, the teacher may say, "Sure, we'll see." This is where you, as the parent, can help. By making that call to the teacher you can let them know you and your child are working on new strategies for success. Once the teacher sees that your child is truly trying to improve they tend to acknowledge the students progress and your child will realize they are indeed improving. Perhaps your child feels they can never do such a thing as ask the teacher to re-explain a particular assignment. Let them know they can ask to speak to the teacher after class. This way they will not feel intimidated or embarrassed in front of their peers. I have never met a teacher unwilling to speak to a student after class when time permits.

Success brings confidence, and once your child begins to see their grades improve and they experience academic success their confidence and self-esteem begin to heighten.

CHAPTER EIGHT

Reward yourself and your child for a job well done. Each time you see success or a glimmer of improvement reward yourself and your child. This can be a simple trip to the coffee shop for their favorite coffee or a stop at the gas station and you pay for the gas that goes in their car, this is providing they normally pay for their own gas. By the way, while I am here, if your teenager drives a car I believe the least, they should do is be paying for the gas to run the car. One parent told me one day that they had really had enough. They actually took the teenagers gas card away. The Mom said, "They will just have to buy their own gas." My question to that mom was, "Why were you buying their gas in the first place?" I do not believe any parent who is reading this book would say, ok, that's it, you are out on the street. Although, sometimes this may be necessary to wake some young people up, depending on their age. Therefore, we want to learn new skills and techniques to ensure this will not occur.

Keep in mind the word responsibility. This reward should be a simple one. No big family dinner out with ballons and candles. We are just experiencing a glimmer of hope here. The war has not been won and I can promise you the battle has just begun.

Just because your child is in high school this does not mean they are now totally responsible for all areas of their life. You do not expect them to buy their own food and prepare it, or pay the utility bills, insurance or mortgage on your home. School is no different. They need to know you are still involved in this area of their lives. There is a comfort in knowing someone is there to check up on them. Believe it or not, teenagers want you to be concerned. They want you to be involved. The secret here is to hit a happy medium and not overpower them. This is where you teach responsibility. Just as with your work you must answer to your boss. If you do not get the job done your boss may call you in to ask if you are having some kind of problems that has prevented you from completing your work. Just letting your child know you care only takes a small amount of effort. Sometimes, it's as simple as asking them how are they doing. When you notice a change in behavior or dedication, they had been showing you can ask them if they are having a problem. Let them know you have noticed a lack of productive behavior with their school work and perhaps even their attitude at home. I highly recommend once you notice a problem address it immediately. Take the time to sit down with your child rather than just in passing by the door to their room and sticking your head in as you are on your way to accomplish another household task.

Your chances of reaching them when you receive their report card and meet them at the door with report card in hand, face red with your temporal veins about to burst, and announce in a very gruff voice, almost a yell that their life, as they know it is over. You're taking the phone, TV, games, and throwing away all those weird clothes they wear. I can only say "Congratulations" you have just hit "0" on the top "10" list. Your child will probably not hear anything you say for the next two days if not weeks. There is a chance your child does not know they have just failed 3 of their 6 classes. On the other hand, they might know. What to do? That is the question. First call them in. Find a quiet place to talk, sit at the kitchen table, or in the den, or wherever the two of you can sit down and have a talk. I would not do this in your bedroom or their bedroom, unless that is the only place to have a quiet conversation. Choose a neutral area, a safe area. Not your turf or theirs, but one that is common to both of you. Do not attack, simply start the conversation with a concerned statement such as "It appears you are still having difficulties in school. Your report card came in the mail, text, or e-mail today." I realize this may seem a little melodramatic. However, your child just failed English, which is, in fact, our spoken language and they have been taking classes in English since kindergarten. They have also failed Physical Education, what is the matter, can't they run, play ball, or jump rope? OK, things are a bit out of control. Take a deep breath and you can deal with this in a controlled manner. You must always remember you are the adult and they are the child. <u>Never, Never, Never</u> let them see you with your boot-straps down when it comes to control. When you have finished the discussion, you may leave the room, go to your bedroom, bury your head in that pillow and scream but you will remain in control while in their presence.

As you begin to discuss the situation with your child, they will undoubtedly begin to explain that that grade was from two weeks ago and they have all "A's" now. In fact, that grade may be two weeks prior, however, it would be the rarest of occasions that the grade has been raised to an "A" in two weeks. Assure your child that you want to believe things are that much better but you will be calling the teachers tomorrow and get a current grade of where they are and discuss with their teachers just what can be done at this point to improve their grades. Secondly, you want to work out a new homework schedule for them so they will begin to see more definite successes. *(Refer to homework plan Chapter Five)*

CHAPTER NINE

These seem to be very simple things to do, however, they are very challenging things to follow through with. When you do follow through you will begin to see improvement. I cannot give you a definite timeline but I can tell you it will be slow and gradual, depending on the severity of the situation you find yourself and your child in. It's like, taking medicine for a serious illness. The condition you are taking the medicine for has been developing over a long period of time and mostly unnoticed. Now you have begun to see symptoms and consulted a doctor. The doctor has prescribed medication which you must take daily. You want to improve so you make sure you are faithful to take the medication daily as prescribed. The same is true for this situation your child is in. This did not happen overnight. The lack of dedication and drive your child has developed is going to take time and immense effort to correct. Trust me, they did not start making "F's" overnight. Perhaps over the past two years or even more. Now you have noticed a steady decline in their grades (job productivity). You kept hoping this was a stage and it would pass without intervention. Now you need intense intervention. Drastic measures sometimes have to be taken in order to see results. This will take an enormous amount of dedication from you and from your child. It will produce good results.

My final words of encouragement come to you from a higher being than any of us. In the book of Job, we find a dedicated man of God who had been stripped of all worldly possessions. He lost the support of his beloved wife and friends. Yet he never failed to remember from where he came. He questioned what had happened to him, he was only human. He did not succumb to the suggestions of his friends and wife to deny God. He remained faithful. In the end he was rewarded with twice as much as he had in the beginning. https://www.i.bible

Good parenting requires collaboration, compromise, tons of love and ten tons of patience. I would suggest to you that you remain strong, stand tall. Your goal is that you will have a cooperative young adult that wants to succeed in life. A teenager that has a desire to learn and reach their maximum potential. This will be the realization of your hard work and their hard work. Determination, and a constant vigil in this process will bring each of you a new and rewarding life.

ABOUT THE AUTHOR

Carolyn Hildebrandt

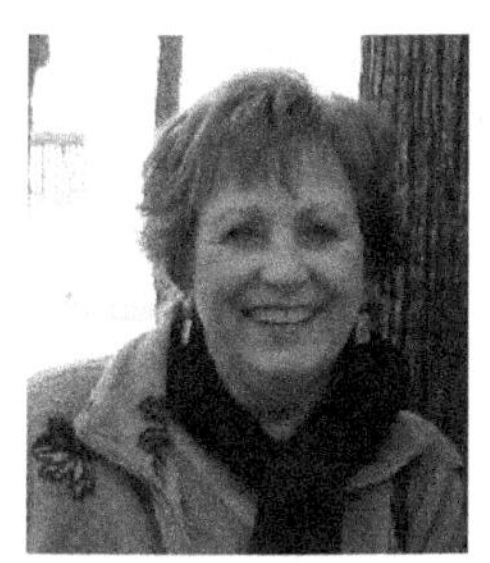 Carolyn is a retired Academic Advisor, Adjunct Professor and Extension Educator. She received her Masters of Psychology from California Coast University and worked as an Academic Advisor for 10 years in the California Public School system. Her experience with students and their parents was extensive and provided most of the skills in the book as a resource she used to ensure students successfully graduated from High School.

Her family moved to Indiana in 2001 where she spent the final eight years of her career. She became an Academic Advisor at Indiana University and Adjunct Professor. There she headed up a program for underprepared students for admission to the University. The goal was to prepare students academically for admission. The program had a 98% success rate. In addition, she was the coordinator of the Special Needs Program at the University. The final leg of her career was with

Purdue University as an Extension Educator. Her interaction with students and their families formed much of her knowledge to direct students and parents into a meaningful, successful life.

Carolyn has two sons who are living successful lives and are now in their 40's. She has one special needs daughter who she navigated through the special Education system. Carolyn and her husband now reside in her home state of Louisiana.

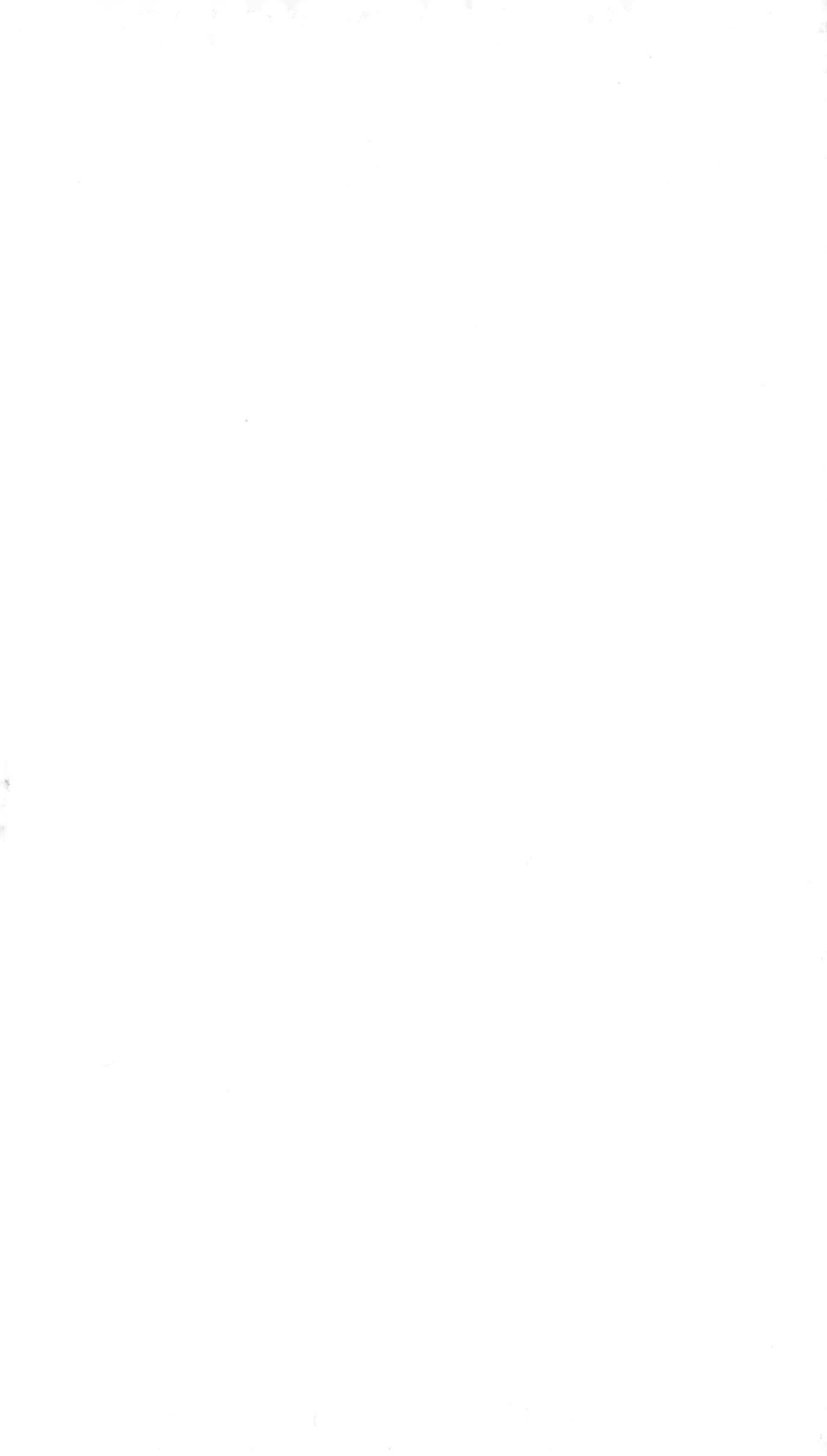